WORK HARD FEEL GOOD

How A Strength Coach Inspires

Athletes For Lifting And Life

Ted Rasmussen

About the Author

Ted Rasmussen owns and operates a private athletic training facility called TNT Strength and Conditioning located in Manahawkin, New Jersey. He is a certified Underground Strength Coach, certified USA Powerlifting Coach and a competitive powerlifter. This coaching facility is designed to help athletes of all sports reach their performance goals.

Here is a message from Coach Ted:

I have been involved with strength training for over 20 years. Having competed from the local to national level for USA Powerlifting, my passion has driven me to help others reach their goals. I have designed and coached strength programs for athletes that participate in a large variety of sports.

Like most young athletes, I have spent a number of misguided years following fads and trends that I would read about in magazines or hear from people in the local gyms. This always left me wondering why my results were not matching my goals. Over time I sought out and learned firsthand from some of the most gifted people in the strength community. Through the teachings from these talented individuals, I learned to apply a never quit work ethic and found the drive to reach my goals and continually set new ones.

TNT is not just a clever name for a strength training company. Each letter represents a name in my family, which serves as a constant reminder to conduct myself with honor and integrity. I do what I do, for my family. As the owner of TNT and the author of this book, I would like to share with you what I have learned, what I teach my athletes, and our motto…WORK HARD FEEL GOOD.

Committed to your success,

Ted Rasmussen

TABLE OF CONTENTS

I BROKE MY BACK

Years ago, I injured my back at my first National Powerlifting Competition. It was not just my lifting that took place at the competition that hurt me, but many things that were leading up to that day. I learned a great deal from this painful experience.

The year was 2010, and I was going through a tremendous amount of stress in my life outside of strength training. My lifting technique was slipping away without me realizing it. I was not under the watchful eye of a coach and I did not have any consistent training partners. The gym I was going to was full of people who were doing more flexing and staring in the mirror and chatting about nonsense, than actually working out. I was surrounded by people who were not experienced in lifting for performance. Needless to say, I was muscling everything up in training instead of dialing in a safe and optimal technique.

Back to the National Competition....I went through my squats feeling okay. The bar slipped down my back on my second attempt, but I was able to successfully go up in weight and make a solid third attempt squat. I went 3 for 3 in the bench press and was looking forward to the deadlift. Deadlifts were always my favorite event to compete in.

After making my first attempt deadlift, I knew it felt heavier than I expected. Still, I went for my planned second attempt and it did not move. I felt a huge deep pain just below my glute on my right leg, and my lower back seemed to lock up. I unsuccessfully tried that weight again on my third attempt. It almost went to full lockout, but I could not complete the lift and I was in pain. This was a 3 times body weight deadlift and looking back at the video of this lift, it was ugly to say the least.

I began training for my next Powerlifting meet practically right away. I was blocking out the pain I was feeling, which really means I was in denial. I did not have my back medically looked at, even though I was at a point where my leg would give out from under me and I would fall doing simple things like stepping over something on the ground or turning around too quickly. It even gave out several times during deadlift training. I was stubborn and had distorted my reality of what was going on.

A few months of painful and frustrating training went by and I was at my next Powerlifting meet in Pennsylvania. This time I "bombed out", which in powerlifting terminology means disqualified. I was unable to do a full squat and failed all 3 attempts. It was a huge let down for me and that's when I snapped out of my tunnel vision and listened to my body.

Prior to that meet, I was negative, close minded and stubborn. Deep down I knew I was hurt but had no one to keep me in check and tell me to back off. Prior to the injury, I had no one to tell me I was lifting incorrectly. I was attacking all my training alone. And most importantly my life was being turned upside down due to personal circumstances. I was recently divorced and a single father learning to raise an amazing toddler. Mental stress can have a huge effect on the body physically but I was naïve to that and learned the hard way.

After that disappointing meet, I refocused my energy to getting better. I was diagnosed with two herniated discs and a third one bulged. They were pushing hard on a root nerve. I found the right doctor who encouraged strength training instead of telling me to give up. I sought out and learned from some of the most talented and successful strength coaches and athletes that I could find. I relearned correct lifting techniques. I also learned that no matter how much experience someone may have, we are all in fact "white belts," needing to constantly reevaluate, learn, and improve. I took my time to get better physically and mentally.

My training program was solid, but now I know and I want to share with you the fact that results are not solely based on the program. It is a combination of many things such as:

Staying stress free as much as possible

Managing stress when it arrives by acknowledging when it arrives and adjusting all things accordingly

Being in the right training environment

Having a great coach

Being positive and optomistc

Not taking things for granted

My most important role here is to be a great coach, to share my knowledge and experiences and help others avoid the mistake that I have made. I am writing this to guide, teach, and most of all, inspire all who read this, to live an awesome strong life.

I hope this helps you on your journey to success.

CHAMPION MINDSET

ALWAYS BE LEARNING

My inspiration for writing this part about learning comes from a powerful weekend that I spent learning to be a better coach by learning to increase my skills to another level. It was spent with coaches with a large variety of skills and experiences. Even with all of that variety, we had a common goal. The quest to continue learning and developing.

I know that I do not have it all figured out. Being aware of this is powerful.

Many coaches do not try to improve. They are "stuck in their ways" and that is an injustice to their athletes. Furthermore, if you are an athlete and are not trying to get better, you are doing an in-justice to your coach, your team, and to yourself. Everyone should always be learning. Even the most highly successful people should not be close minded in thinking that they can't learn anymore. We can all learn more.

The greatest champions of all time became champions because they know that each day the training starts over with new knowledge. New knowledge from both study and experience. Sometimes we relearn what we once knew and other times we learn new things, but either way we all must realize that we do not know it all and do not have it all figured out.

If you continue to learn, you will continue to improve. With that approach towards growth and development, you can do anything in life.

IT IS NOT GOING TO BE EASY

Athletes cannot cut corners, and short cuts are not an option. At the end of the day, you know if you did exactly what you needed to do. Be honest with yourself.

Be accountable to yourself.

It is not always going to be fun. There are times when you may want to quit, when you doubt yourself, when your goals seem to be slipping away. This is normal. It is part of the process. The Ultimate Warrior referred to this as "Mr. Resistance."

Do not let the resistance win. Fight back! Stand up to the challenges. Embrace the hard times, your work ethic will get you through. Our bodies can do much more than our minds allow us to believe!

Be a warrior!

Strength training is a skill. You cannot just go through the motions and expect to have results. You must be consistent, but showing up is not good enough!! **Put forth your best effort the whole time, every time!**

DON'T COMPETE

It seems to be a growing trend to tell our youth not to compete. That everyone should get a turn and a reward. Many people in society do not encourage competition.

People who are in a position to really change lives for the better such as teachers, role models, and several other highly influential people, have literally said, "Don't compete. It's not fair to everyone else." They shy away from friendly competition in exchange for some sort of collective fairness.

This teaches someone to not challenge themselves nor challenge others for personal growth, in fear that someone may get their feelings hurt. Fear that a line will be drawn showing a winner on one side and a loser on the other. There seems to be more and more people thinking everyone should get a trophy regardless of who is actually the best.

In my opinion that way of thinking is weak, plain and simple. In today's world, having a competitive spirit is crucial to achieving success. Be it in sport, school, or your job, meritocracy is not a bad thing, it's a must!

When there is competition, good ideas turn into great ideas, average athletes turn into highly successful athletes, and employees begin to operate in such a motivated fashion they go above the so called "job description"

The mind switches gears and that's when things can really take off. That's where the competitive spirit lives, in the minds of motivated successful people.

When competition does not exist or is removed from the situation, being average becomes the "normal." Average is safe and comfortable. It is the easy path. Being competitive pushes you out of your comfort zone. I would never want to settle for being average. I would much rather fail knowing that I tried my absolute best and earned a place below first, than to take the easy way out.

No one can be great at everything but everyone can be great at something. To be great, you have to push the limits and risk exposing failure. A lot can be learned from failure. With great risk comes great reward.

CAN WE DARE TO BE GREAT

At **TNT Strength and Conditioning**, everyone works hard, they always do. The athletes set examples to those around us. We do not train to be average. We train to be great.

Greatness does not fall into your lap, you need to push yourself to achieve greatness. Opportunities may fall into your lap, but if you do not follow though, the opportunity is gone.

I have watched our crew inspire each other to work for greatness, and they inspire me big time. As I change their lives, they change mine.

At **TNT**, we are a family..... a strong family who pushes, encourages, and supports one another.

To achieve greatness in life, you better be prepared to struggle, to strain hard and push the envelope. Anyone who has inspired and changed the world did so by not being average. They shut out the naysayers and dared themselves to be great!

WHEN A LEADER FAILS

I remember training in my garage gym as I was preparing for a National Powerlifting Competition. The garage was cold as it always was in the winter, but I was fired up to put in the work. A few of my student athletes were watching and that was a great motivator. It was deadlift day and the prescription called for a one rep max effort with as much weight as I could handle and four 5/8" chains on the bar as well.

As I warmed up and started working my way up in weight towards that one rep max, things were feeling and moving well. I knew it was time for a new personal record. I asked one of the spectating athletes to record the lift. I would use that video to review my technique plus it also meant they would be closely watching. I remember thinking, "I better not miss this one. My students are watching and that camera is on."

I got psyched up and ready to go. Set up my stance, grabbed the bar, and began to pull. It felt heavy. And guess what happened next…I missed the lift. I couldn't get the bar above my knees. Those 5/8" chains started loading up and I was stuck.

My athletes were disappointed and I was too. I was not about to walk away like that. I could have called it quits, but no way. That's not what I teach them and that is not how I live my life. I do not like losing. If you want to win you must hate losing.

I told them, "I'm going to do this again."

They doubted me and said that I was crazy, but I believed in myself. Even if I am crazy to try again, I was determined. Now I had something to prove to them and more importantly, to me.

I chalked my hands, tightened my power belt, found some of that inner fire, took a deep breath and pulled that chain filled bar all the way to lock out. When the bar got to my knees, it was just a check point. A check point to not give up.

Overcoming a heavy deadlift has a unique and awesome feeling. At the moment I stood straight up with my face bright red (as seen on the video) and knees locked out, everyone in the garage learned something. We collectively learned that failure is not an option and ones mindset must recognize this.

I came back to the challenge and got the job done. I knew what I was capable of, made the necessary technique adjustments, and executed. This type of refocusing is something we are all capable of. Learn from your failures and try again.

If we are to complete the task at hand, whatever that may be, we must attack it with everything we have inside.

The important lesson here, and possibly the most important lesson for me to teach my athletes, is to always believe in yourself.

WINNING ISN'T EVERYTHING!!

Winning isn't everything but it sure does feel good to win. True competitors do not train to be second best. They do not play to lose.

Losing is part of every sport. Losing is part of life. A lot can be learned when you lose. I don't encourage being a sore loser. Win or lose, we all need to remain respectful, but to get to the top you have to hate losing. You must want more than just being average. Average may be good enough for some coaches, but it's not what I want to represent. I believe in taking a stand and doing great things. I want to see people going above the average. This is hard to do but it's within the hard times that the true champions live.

You should attack life with this mindset by putting in your best effort with all the things that you do. Learn from your mistakes. Learn from when you lose. Push forward and become a champion. Which is not always measured in trophies, it is measured by work ethic and determination.

WHAT REALLY MATTERS

Getting results matter. Loving that process is the best part. When you put in the hard work and make it part of your life, you will get the real results. That's what matters, working and achieving your goals.

When it comes to working out, the trendy do not care about the results. Companies and influencers pitch to you the greatest machine or diets, making you feel like its easy and comfortable.

Don't be fooled by the shortcuts and gimmicks that are out there. There are no shortcuts when you want real results. There is only hard work, dedication, consistency, and a lifetime of accomplishing small goals.

It's in our motto**...**" **Work Hard, Feel Good"**

STEP UP TO NEW CHALLENGES

Living an awesome life is not always easy. It's not always going to feel like a walk in the park on a warm sunny day. Often times it feels like the opposite. This happens because life puts up road blocks.

But if you look at the road blocks as stepping stones, and face your fears, and conquer the challenges, you will learn a great deal about yourself and what you are capable of doing.

It is my belief that we can all do anything as long as we dedicate the time and effort to figuring it out.

Facing ones fears is a very hard thing to do. Often when you fear trying new things, it's much easier to give in and walk the other way. This is a weak way of thinking. It's a mindset that everyone struggles with. Step up to the challenge and you will find reward. Personal growth happens when we overcome a challenge.

If you are trying a new sport or position in your current sport or job, don't back down. Stand up to the challenge and work.

If you have never jumped off of a diving board, walk up to the thing and jump! If you have never flipped over a tractor tire, try it. It may end up being your favorite training tool.

The point is this, be strong in all aspects of your life.

LIVING WITH PASSION

One thing that has always been a staple in my life is passion. I have always lived my life in a passionate way. I do not believe in doing things halfway. To me, it will always be all in.

Sometimes my passionate way of speaking has been interpreted as aggression. When I am fired up about something, I don't sit quietly, but my passion should not be confused with anger or negativity.

To me life should be lived in a passionate way. Going through life in a very bland and mundane way is a waste of time. One thing we all have in common is time and that can never be re-wound.

As we get older, our likes, interests, and hobbies change.The things we used to love to do may no longer seem fun or a big deal anymore. That's okay, but whatever you are engaged in, be it your job, your sport, whatever, do it with passion.

HAVING THE RIGHT ATTITUDE

Achieving your goals...Not settling for average...Being the best that you can be...These are all very important statements. At their very core, they are a big part of what makes up feeling good from putting in the hard work.

I often talk about these things with our members at TNT. It's a positive message and that is what we represent here. Working hard and feeling good for it. Sometimes this message is misunderstood.

Everyone is different and will have different values and different goals. Some people do not really have goals. We are all unique. I want everyone to strive to be the best that they can be. I also believe that we should not put people down or make them feel inferior because they don't attack their life goals the same way that others do.

We train hard. It makes us stronger both physically and mentally. Athletes are competitive. It's in our nature, but not everyone is an athlete. Not everyone cares about what we do. Not everyone will care about what you do. I don't want anyone reading this to think that they are up on some pedestal, being better than those who are different and have different interests and values.

Many things in life are out of our control but what you can control is yourself. Living a strong way of life comes down to having the right attitude and knowing that you are doing what you need to do and not wasting time hating on others. You will develop confidence from strength training. Never make the mistake and exchange your confidence for arrogance.

You do not have to have a special talent to be in control of yourself. Here are just a few things that you can control right now without any specific skills or education.

Be nice to others even if they are different

Be the hardest worker in the room

Show up early, stay late and work

Put in extra credit

Share your knowledge

Inspire others and lead by example

GOALS

GOALS

Goal setting is SUPER important. You must have small goals AND big goals.

The small goals, that you are not too far away from reaching, will keep you motivated and confident.

The big goals, the ones that seem so far away you start thinking they might never happen, they keep you working. Keep the desires burning! One must never settle for just being satisfied.

"Satisfaction is the death of desire."-Jamey Jasta

If you get stuck and cannot figure out how to get to the "next level," how to reach that goal that seems so impossible right now, the best piece of advice that I can offer is to PAY ATTENTION. Trust yourself and pay attention to your instincts. Pay attention to your surroundings. Most of the time, the answers are right in front of you.

We can all reach our goals if we put in the time and effort to achieve them. Simply put, be committed to your own success.

THE MESSAGE TODAY IS.....

Surround yourself with a group of positive individuals who are attacking life with the same relentless pursuit that you are. Our goals are our own. So is our ability to learn and apply that knowledge. The hard work and effort that we put in is also our own, but we are not alone.

There are people out in the world who are motivated and hard working even if you can't see them. People with goals and a game plan for making it happen. Sometimes you have to just avoid negative people to find them. The one's who don't believe in your vision or are turned off by your passion.

Surround yourself with likeminded people. Seek out individuals who are also setting their own goals and putting in their best effort to achieve those goals. Being around successful and motivated people has a power that is hard to put into words. They can keep you pushing for more when you want to quit and you can inspire those around you to push for more when they want to quit. It makes challenging times fun when we are all in it together for the greater good of self improvement.

ANOTHER MONDAY!

I hope that you are not one of the "regular people" who hate Mondays. I personally want to love Monday as much as any other day of the week. I have a lot of Mondays left in me and I want to make the most out of ALL of them.

Going back to school or work or whatever you are engaged in is not always easy after a few days off. After a break from the "routine" it can become hard to find inspiration to enjoy the "daily grind."

When this happens I want you to think about your goals. Realize that you have the ability and the tools to do great things. There is no doubt in my mind that you do not have inspiration all around you. When you open your mind and look around you will find it. Even on a Monday.

WHAT DOES IT TAKE?

How do you define success? Once you have that figured out, how do you achieve that success? Will you be committed to take the necessary steps or are you just dreaming?

You should be asking yourself these questions often. Your answers will most likely be very different from mine or anyone else really. That's okay. It's your success and not theirs.

Training is much more than the weight room and your sport. The lessons learned during competitive training can be applied to all aspects of your life and not just to your sport. You lean that you are the one who is responsible for reaching your goals. You also learn how to push through these really difficult times when the odds are stacked up against you and things become a mental challenge just as much if not more than the physical. When you are dedicated you lean a tremendous amount about who you are and what you are capable of.

Define your success. Dedicate yourself to achieving it, AKA, do the work! I promise in the end you will not be disappointed.

BREAKING HABITS TO REACH YOUR GOALS

Most people have a routine. You wake up at a certain time each day. You get ready for the day in a fairly specific way. It's your morning routine. Many of you go through the day following a daily routine. It's very safe and comfortable.

I want to challenge you to step outside of that habit. I want you to do something that makes you uncomfortable. I am not saying do something negative. It has to be of a positive benefit to your life and/or someone else's. "Get comfortable being uncomfortable." I'm not sure who said it first, but the first time I heard this was from my friend Zach Even-Esh and it has stuck with me ever since.

I hope by now you are inspired to have more out of life than just average. I hope that you want to live a great life!

The way to achieve that great life is not easy. It requires hard work and dedication. When you can learn to break through your safe zone, break the daily routine and do the things that need to be done regardless of how uncomfortable that may be, you will begin to find new success.

Think about what it will take to reach your goals. To accomplish those things in life that you feel are important.

Do you have a plan? Are you taking the necessary steps to execute that plan, or are you going through life with a daily routine that does not dare you to challenge yourself? Break away from those habits that are keeping you from living the life you deserve.

FACE THE CHALLENGES

There is a great feeling of reward when you set your sites on a challenging goal and you put forth real effort to accomplish it. To achieve this, you must learn to have a love and a passion for the hard work. A love for the challenge. If you fear the challenge, then that fear will stand in your way. Do not let anything stand in your way.

I love strength training. I love the hard work and the challenge that comes with it. This can be extremely uncomfortable, but it's what I live for. I also love the feeling of getting better at everyday life through strength training.

My real passion and purpose is to be able to share this hard work with athletes. To offer my coaching to others and watch them develop and become better at what they love and better at living a strong life. This requires me and them to face challenges.

I believe that we all have the ability to do great things within our lives. It is my mission to impact lives in a positive way. This holds true for my family, for all of the athletes who put their trust in me, and for you reading this book.

TRAINING

TRAINING WITH AGGRESSION

The bar is loaded. On the floor of my garage gym sits a pile of iron, waiting for me. The music is cranking my favorite deadlift song, **"Make War, Not Love" by Pro-Pain.**

I chalk my hands, tighten my wrist wraps and lock in my belt. I'm ready to rip it off of the floor.

As I approach the bar, my mind starts thinking. Thinking about technique...Thinking about past injuries...I want to make sure that everything is perfect. I set up my feet, lift my arms up, and take in a big breath of air, and brace my abs. I stay in a tightly locked position. All the while I'm thinking about every inch of movement. Asking myself, "Am I staying tight? Are my back and shoulders in the right position?" I feel the bar and tighten my grip. It's time to lift it. And what happens? ...It doesn't move. It feels impossible.

I cannot believe it went nowhere!

I step back and realize what went wrong. With all of the thoughts making the set up perfect, all the mental cues running through my head, I forgot a very important thing…..aggression. Heavy weight will not move if you do not use your inner fire! Aggression, adrenaline, and speed, will help get things going. It's mental toughness, a skill that must be practiced. Without it you may find yourself feeling weak.

Learn to be aggressive with your training. This goes for high rep sets too. When fatigue starts to set in and you are not done with your set, training with aggression will get you there.

Heavy weights and hard challenging sets cannot be approached without an aggressive attack. This does not mean that you have to "burn yourself out" by getting overly psyched up, but you better be ready to bring it!

Methodical lifting is good with lighter weights. It teaches you form and technique. You learn the motor patterns of the lift and develop habits.

Habits cannot be thought about when it is go time. It must be second nature.

When I smash a P.R. (personal record), what goes through my mind as I set up and execute? Nothing. My mind is blank, but my focus and intensity are cranked way up. Sometimes we need to silence out inner voices and just get it done!

THE POWER OF BODYWEIGHT TRAINING

Learn how to make great progress using just your body. Body weight only exercises will make you strong and athletic. Many people think unless you are lifting weights, you can't get strong and build muscle.

Now don't get me wrong, I love lifting weights. Heavy cold steel is awesome. After all, I do coach the sport of Powerlifting!

One should never underestimate the raw power of body weight training. All athletes need to develop and possess coordination, strength, speed, and power. All of this can be accomplished by using your body and not machines or weights. This type of training will also provide conditioning, muscle building, and fat loss.

I have put this type of training to the test for myself and our athletes. This is a no gimmicks approach. Believe me, we are not exercising with a ripped model "as seen on TV.: We are straight up, "Bodyweight Body Building," which is the name of a great program to check out by Zach Even-Esh.

Our training programs always include bodyweight work. It's simple, basic, hard, and gets the job done.

Is it popular to say things are basic or hard? No, but we do not train to be popular. We train to get results.

The hard work is what does it and not the short cuts.

TNT PROGRAM DESIGN

Most of my athletic development programming is based on the fundamentals of the concurrent system. I will mix between full body days and days focusing on upper and lower. The workouts are typically programmed for 3-4 week waves and the intent is this:

Week 1: introduce the movements and establish a base with the weights, reps, and flow of the workout

Week 2: improve from week 1, either with technique, weight being used, or both

Week 3&4: hit a personal record (P.R.) with weight, reps, or time, depending on the specifics of the workout

Let me further explain what the concurrent system if training is. This system uses the approach of blending together multiple strength skills within each workout phase. An athlete would con- sistently work on strength, power, muscle building, endurance, and conditioning as opposed to having an individual "block" where each skill is worked on separately, moving from one skill to the next after the block (typically 3-4 weeks) is complete.

Depending on what each individual needs, the concurrent system allows the main focus to be adjusted to the athletes needs while still working on, or maintaining the other strength skills.

The training and development of athletes cannot always be approached with a specific phase or time period (block) devoted to one strength skill at a time. Athletes are extremely busy going to practices, private club training, games, and tournaments. They have schedules that are all over the place and this puts their bodies and minds through a lot of stress. It also leads to missing workouts during the preseason and in season or at the very least allowing less available time to work out within a session.

This is why this style of training works great for the training of sport athletes. It allows us to work on general physical preparation year round and the ability to adjust any of the strength skills or conditioning as needed without getting too far away from any one attribute.

Athletes of any sport need to be strong, fast, powerful/explosive, and to be able to have the strength endurance to maintain a high level of athleticism for an entire game, match, or meet.

TRAINING TIPS

Here I am going to share with you some basic training principles that can be applied right now. Whether you are designing training programs or doing the workouts yourself, these training tips can help and are listed in no particular order.

-Allow For Recovery Between Sets-

Apply this to free weight training, sprints, and high intensity circuits. This could mean up to 3 minutes of rest before doing you next set. Allow for your breathing and heart rate to return to or close to a normal pace. Many people do this for their heavy weight training but then rush through their sprints or high intensity work. Moving fast between sets will increase your endurance but when maximal force output is the goal, rest before you explode.

-Keep Your Body Tight-

Keep your entire body tight when performing static single plane power movements. By bracing your body you are able to support the heavy loads, maintain proper posture, and recruit the maximum amount of muscle fibers.

-Work on Your Weaknesses-

Heavy weights will expose where you are weak. Your performance is only as strong as that weak link. For example, your legs may be strong enough to squat a certain weight, but if your abdominals cannot support it then you do not squat it. Train what you are good at to maintain and improve skill and stay confident. Train your weak areas, to guarantee that you get better.

-Include All Types of Strength Skills-

A solid program must blend MAXIMUM EFFORT (moving heavy loads), DYNAMIC EFFORT (speed/power), and REPETITION EFFORT (muscle building and strength endurance). Performance improves when these speed skills improve.

Explosive Strength=FAST speed

(explosive/dynamic)- Jump training/plyometric

Speed Strength=INTERMEDIATE speed

(dynamic)- Acceleration at maximum velocity with sub-maximal resistance

Strength Speed=SLOWER speed

(max)- Ability to overcome large amounts of resistance

You must leave no stone unturned when designing and performing a training program for athletes.

WHAT IS ALL THIS CONDITIONING TALK?

Over the years, I have received a fair amount of questions about the conditioning part of our program. So I want to take a few moments of your time to clear some things up.

Conditioning can be approached in many ways but I will break it down into two types: Specific and General.

Specific conditioning is used to physically prepare you for a certain event or activity. A conditioning program for a wrestler or an MMA fighter would look quite different from that of a power-lifter or a baseball player. It's a calculated program that closely resembles the sport.

General conditioning is used to bring up your physical fitness to whatever level is necessary to stay healthy and allow you to increase your training work capacity. This would be your baseline that you develop throughout the year.

Either way the point of training to increase your conditioning is NOT to leave piles of puke on the floor or even worse, get hurt. Conditioning should do the opposite. It should be preventing injuries by an increased GPP (General Physical Preparedness).

I train athletes so we adjust the amount of specific conditioning based on the time of year and their sport. I also adjust it based on the current level of their general fitness/athletic capabilities. This is the art of coaching.

In the "off" season, the focus is more strength based or muscle building with the conditioning portion designed to aid in building strength. As they approach the "in" season, the conditioning begins to increase towards the specifics for their sport.

The conditioning is cycled and can be programmed similar to cycling strength blocks. Ramp it up and then back it down while adjusting the workout accordingly. This keeps athletes physically healthy and prevents mental burnout.

Athletes all have different levels of what they can recover from and what they need to develop. Some may be able to do conditioning work for a large number of minutes straight during a workout while others may only be able to handle a few minutes. Intensity has a lot to do with that as well, and should be adjusted based on the individual.

IN Season vs OFF Season

Training is done year round. Consistency is a key part to reaching your goals. The off season training is very important to not just make gains but to allow your body to properly recover from the demands placed upon it during the competitive sport. Grow and develop in the OFF season and the IN season. You cannot just stop your strength program because you are participating in a sport and/or sport practice.

For the purpose of this chapter, I'm referring to competitive athletes but please keep in mind that this also applies to non athletes as well. Just because life's chores or your tasks at your job ramp up and make getting to the gym harder, you should not use that as an excuse to stop working on your fitness all together.

Moving on, let's put together a hypothetical scenario that is very common for developing athletes. You have been strength training hard and consistent for 4 months. You have been making gains physically and mentally. You're stronger, more conditioned, and more confident than ever before. Now after 4 months, your team begins to practice. Your games begin and you're getting good playing time. You have to study and do homework. You decide to stop working out, thinking how the last 4 months will carry over.

I have seen this type of thing happen over and over again and this is what it leads to.

You will go into your preseason sport training looking like a whole new athlete. The coaches and spectators will be like, "Wow! What have you been doing?!" As the season progresses and since your strength training has come to a halt, you will begin to slow down, get weaker, and you may lose your confidence to some degree. As you get through the season, and get to the most important part of your sport, playoffs, big tournaments, finals, etc., you will actually be worse from an athletic stand point than when you started. One can only hope that everyone else has stopped training and are following suit just like you.

In season training is vital to keeping you strong, healthy, and maintaining the best possibility to be injury free. Of course your sports specific practice becomes priority, but your strength and general conditioning need to be on point during the in season.

As a side note, competing in strength sports, like powerlifting during an athletes' off season is a fantastic way to keep technique dialed in, giving training a competitive feel with goals and a deadline to achieve said goals. It creates an "in season" feel to your sports "off season." Something I feel athletes should strongly consider.

UNDERSTANDING THE BOX SQUAT

Box squats are an excellent and safe way to improve not just you squat but your overall strength. Low box squats (below parallel) put you in the right spot for optimal performance and teach your body to learn where below parallel actually is. High box squats can help you work through specific ranges of motion in the squat.

These can be used by the novice lifter or the advanced. Some people fear that squatting on a box is bad for the back. That is incorrect. They are safe, like anything else, if performed properly. Poor technique in any exercise can lead to injury.

The two biggest mistakes that I see people make when box squatting is:

Crashing down onto the box

Relaxing when they reach the box

These things can easily be corrected with proper coaching and I am here to help. If you are crashing down, you must control your body better. This is usually a case of weak hamstrings. The solution is to work your hamstrings harder. To quickly build them up, add in extra hamstring specific work such as band leg curls. Do these on the day(s) you train your lower half as well as on your "off" days.

As for relaxing on the box, most athletes do not even realize that they are doing it. Here is a solution to help prevent this from happening. When you completely reach the box (hamstrings and glutes are in complete contact), your feet must be firmly planted to the ground. You must remain tight. If someone can walk over to you and kick your feet away or you are wiggling around, you are not tight. Just because you are sitting down, does not mean that you lose body tightness and awareness. We are not watching T.V., we are squatting!

Here is how a box squat is executed:

Get tight (everywhere).......Sit back, not straight down

Stay tight·.....Release your hips so you can touch the box (DO NOT BE RELAXED)

Explode back up as fast and as forceful as possible leading with the bar up and not your hips.

Include box squats in your training and the amount of weight you can squat will increase, your performance will improve, and your confidence will go up.

TRAINING WITH PAIN

What do you do when you have an ach or pain that will not go away? Or even worse, a diagnosed injury?

Do you completely stop training and risk losing all the gains you have worked so hard for? If that's what you do, I want you to know that there is another way.

Training with an injury is not always fun. It requires you to be more cautious and calculated with things within your training that you are not used to thinking about.

You may have heard or even been told to stop working out when you are injured. Well, I do not subscribe to this school of thought. There are things you can do.

There is always a way to train around the injured area without getting hurt or slowing down your recovery.

For example, you lower back hurts so you train arms and chest. You may not be able to squat, deadlift, and do bent over rows, but try doing things like seated hammer curls, lying tricep extensions, seated shoulder presses, lateral raises, and band pull aparts. Maybe you have been neglecting your grip strength. I'm pretty sure even with a herniated disc you could find a way to get in some dumbbell hex holds or gripper work. It's a matter of trial and error.

I am not a doctor so this advice is really just from my experiences. Throughout my life I have seen injured people safely train and train hard. Even with a broken leg in a cast. This obviously complicates things but by no means do you have to completely stop your training.

I have seen people paralyzed from the waist down set world records in the bench press, a blind athlete win big wrestling tournaments, and I have even worked out side by side with an individual in a wheel chair. Although he couldn't squat and lunge, there was plenty he could do. It inspires me big time when I think about it.

The worst thing to do is give up on your physical training. Not only does this negatively affect your body, but it has a negative effect on your mind. I am telling you this with firsthand experience. Your body and your mind will be much more happy when you are training and not lying around feeling sorry for yourself.

OUR GYM'S STANDARD

The standard for most places is a baseline showing what the minimum level of acceptance is. Some facilities or clubs may want to see a certain weight one can lift or a particular time one can reach in a drill. Maybe it's a certain level someone has reached or record they have set.

When I thing about what our standard is at TNT, I can guarantee that the standard we uphold is a standard of excellence.

I look at it like this….. if you are not pursuing excellence, then to put it bluntly, you don't belong with us. We are a performance based training facility and I do not just let thing slide. Laziness is not tolerated and drama is not welcome. Saying that you're good enough is not accepted. Training with me is about sports and life. We learn to push through difficult times so you can live a great life. Both in and out of the athletic arena.

Some coaches will take it easy, sit back and allow things that are far short of excellence to be accepted. To them, being good enough is okay.

I want everyone that I coach to strive for something great. To strive for something more than the short term goal. From a novice to a highly advanced athlete, the standard is equal and that standard is excellence. No matter where you train or what you are doing uphold that standard in everything that you do.

NO MIRRORS

I do not have mirrors in my gym for people to watch themselves train. If you need to watch yourself to see if you are doing the movement correctly, you will not develop the correct motor skills to master it.

I love the squat so let's use that as an example. Many gyms have a full body mirror in front of the power rack or squat stands. I think it can be quite dangerous to be staring at down at yourself during a squat workout. If you need to check your depth or see if your knees are caving in, how focused are you? Your visual needs to be a blur if you are to truly execute at your best level. Not staring down at your knees.

That's my job as the coach at a coaching facility. I watch everyone's form and we constantly work on technique. I know that there are coaches who do not pay close attention to the details, but that's not me. I also know that sport coaches try to be the strength coach in many schools. I'm sure some are good, but many just don't know what to look for. I don't teach athletes how to run a football drill, pitch a curveball, or do double leg take downs. That is not my skill set. Just as proper lifting technique and programming is not theirs.

Anyway back to mirrors. Commercial gyms have mirrors because people love to look at themselves. Go on social media and you will see a lot more selfies before you find the useful information. Watching yourself workout and getting pumped up can elevate you confidence for sure, but in sports, you can't watch yourself like that. Unless you are a body builder or physique competitor monitoring your actual appearance to track visual progress, you don't need a mirror during a workout.

It's my belief that athletes need to feel the movement. They need the physical cues that the body gives to know if they are doing something correctly. Videos can be very helpful to assess form and technique after you have completed the lift. Mirrors are distractions. Stay focused on lifting correctly and check yourself in the mirror before you leave the bathroom.

DO THE WORK

TIME IS PRECIOUS

Time is precious and it is tricky. Five years from now feels like you have all the time in the world. It seems far away. Five years ago can feel like it just happened. Like where did all of that time go?

Life goes by fast. To me it seems like it was not that long ago that I was a kid playing G.I. Joes with my friends. Although my son is grown and is now taller than me, it feels like I was just holding his hand in parking lots yesterday.

Our window of opportunity can be very small. If you spend your life waiting to get things done instead of taking immediate action it could very well be too late. Having the ability to work hard is a privilege. There will come a day when you will not be able to be so active. Spending you life wasting time is a tragic mistake. I suggest that you take time to thank those who have helped inspire you and to help inspire those who need you. But most importantly, take action on whatever it is that you want to do. You know that thing that you dream of or the thing that you keep putting off waiting for the "right time." Well that right time is now.

HOW BAD DO YOU WANT IT?

Every overnight success probably has a long back story that you never hear about. To be successful, you must attack the necessary work and continue to attack.

You cannot have everything right away. You must put in the time and the work. Many people waste time over thinking their strategy to success. The one thing we can all do is also the most over looked and least talked about. This is consistency. It's a basic principle to achieving success, but it's also one of the hardest. Being consistent requires real mental toughness. Anyone can start something, but it takes a certain discipline to stick with it. This applies to nutrition, exercise, and really all aspects of life.

You have to consistently follow the diet to be healthy. You have to continually work hard in the gym to build up your body. You have to consistently strive to be a better person. You can't just do it when it's convenient and easy, you must do it when it takes everything that you've got, to stick with the plan.

Putting in the work for just a short period of time will give you short lived results. Putting in the work every month, every week, and every day, will give you a life time of feeling and being successful.

THE IMPORTANCE OF TEAMWORK

Team work is excellent. Watching our athletes work as a team while doing their own individual work is just awesome.

The energy is high and the atmosphere is positive. They are not only developing strength but they are also developing a positive attitude. Both of which will last a lifetime.

After coaching our workouts, I am energized and excited to crush my own training. I feel ready to be the leader of my team. Not simply the instructor but someone who is going through it just like they are.

If you are not part of a "team," I suggest you be part of something. Some type of community that will motivate you and help keep you accountable. You need to do things on your own, but you are NOT alone. Like-minded people are out there. We can all be in this together!

LEAD BY EXAMPLE

Today I talked myself out of doing my scheduled training session at least 5 times. I would make an excuse in my mind and try to settle on the fact that I was going to miss my work out.

I was telling myself things like.............

"I'm still sore from the last workout."

"I can skip today and make it up during the week."

"I didn't sleep well or eat well, so the workout will not be good anyway."

The bottom line is that I was making excuses. I was talking myself out of doing something that is a positive benefit to improving the quality of my life.

Then I started thinking about my son, and all of the athletes I have worked with, I was thinking how hard they work. How I would never let them tell me the things that I was telling myself. If they knew that I missed workouts because I was making lazy excuses, they would lose respect for me and it would give them the green light to give into their own excuses.

So I hardened up, got the tunes cranking, and had a killer TNT style workout.

As a father, a coach, and a competitive athlete, I lead by example. You should too.

FANCY TOOLS AND SMILING FACES

I distinctly remember being in a gym that is owned by one of the local hospitals here in my area of southern N.J. This gym was called a Life Center and it had "everything." A staff that included chiropractors, personal trainers, physical therapists, and massage therapists, equipment such as plyometric boxes of all sizes, kettle bells, dumbbells over 120 lbs, Hammer Strength power racks, multiple benches, specialty bars, ropes for climbing and slams, tractor tires, every machine you could think of, and an indoor track. There were rooms for cardio, free weights, aerobics, and combat training with heavy bags and speed bags for punching. I'm sure I am forgetting to list a few things, but the point is, this place had all the "tools" you could think of.

The one huge important thing it did not have was people working out hard. Among all of this equipment, was a dead environment. No one was breaking a sweat. I saw members doing paperwork on the benches. The trainers were all having casual conversations with their clients while they were "working out." Everyone was chatting and sharing stories. The physical therapists and massage therapists seemed to be the only ones actually focused and working.

Something hit me hard when I was in there. It's part of the fitness industry that does not resonate with me. You see, people get sold on the gimmicks and flashy training tools. They get sold on the idea that the place has everything that they need, like somehow that's enough to reach their goals.

It's not all the functional training equipment, multiple personal trainers on hand, or any of those types of things that will get you where you want to get. Can that stuff help? Of course it can. I use a lot of that equipment for my athletes and for myself but the most important thing you need and what's not talked about by fitness industry salesman is dedication. Dedication and a will to push yourself for excellence.

That mindset and dedication will always out do all of those other things. I know for a fact that you can have better results with zero equipment, training in your bedroom with bodyweight only workouts as opposed to slacking off with the fancy equipment surrounding you.

The equipment doesn't do the work for you, nor does the personal trainer or the gym. You do the work for you. The fitness industry sells people on hope with false promises. Too many, trainers view what they do as just a job instead of realizing the opportunity they have to change people's lives. The bottom line is this....if you want results, do the work...it is that simple!

DON'T BE SO CONFUSED

There is way too much confusion when it comes to strength training. The internet is full of all of these so called fitness gurus who have the latest and greatest program for you to follow. Social media is flooded with people using fancy terms to trick you into making a purchase. They offer short cuts and gimmicky exercises that look great on a YouTube video.

"6 Minutes to 6 Pack abs"

"Train Your Anterior Core"

"Football Specific Workouts" (or any sport)

"Short Cuts to Your Success"

The list goes on and on and the sad part is that people buy into this stuff without realizing what it really takes to be successful and make gains in your training.

Hard work.....Attack the basics

Master Technique

Commitment to training, nutrition, and recovery

Be early and stay late….Do extra

Don't make excuses

This list goes on and on as well.

Someone selling immediate success is not telling you the whole story, which is it will most likely not last. The truth is it's a lifetime of commitment. That may not be the popular thing to say, but you can bet it's the truth. The best of the best spend years getting better.

There is no quick fix when it comes to finding and mastering who you are and all of the great things that you have to offer.

I do not have all of the answers, but what I do have is a community of professionals with common goals. They offer their personal experiences and expertise to help change the lives of others. To these people it is not just about the money, it's about sharing and providing useful information. Sort through the confusion and find yourself a community in which you can lean and thrive in.

STAY ON COURSE

What do you do when times are hard? Do you find another path and take the easy route? Do you make excuses that hold you back from overcoming the hard times? Or do you stay on course?

My inspiration for writing this comes from a conversation that I had with a friend one weekend. We spoke of people we knew who began doing awesome and positive things in their life, but backed away as soon as they faced adversity. They called it quits when things got difficult. It reminded me just how important it is to stay committed even when the lines get blurred and things become a challenge.

We all go through difficult times. Some are much harder than others. When you are stuck in that moment I know it's hard to push through. The easy choice is not always the right choice.

I have faced very challenging situations in my personal life. Just like many of you. What gets me through those times is my commitment to better myself.

This is not just about exercising; it's about living a great life. You must learn to be true to who you are. Don't fail yourself. Learn to stay on course, to stay on YOUR course.

"When I make a commitment, I stay true to what is right. I will never make a commitment unless it's for life." –Roger Miret

DOING EXTRA WORK

We have all experienced times where it is super hard to get motivated. We find ourselves procrastinating. I remember one time in particular that I would like to share.

It was an evening in the spring. The weather was warming up here in New Jersey and the sun was staying out longer. I was tired and wanted to go to sleep. I knew that if I sat down and closed my eyes I would be out.

I was feeling slow, lazy, and basically unhappy with myself. I was second guessing my strength and even my capabilities to ever get better. My training focus was powerlifting and chasing numbers on the bar can really mess with ones mindset.

I started to think about my passion. I began to feel it deep inside. I kicked the negative thoughts right out of my head and found my inspiration from within. I was inspired by my own desire to get better.

This was an "off" day from my training program but I knew I needed to do some work to start feeling better. To find that part of myself I am proud of. It was a perfect time to add in extra work.

Extra workouts or mini workouts are used to increase you general preparedness and heighten your mental awareness. These are short workouts that increase your heart rate but are done at a low intensity. These workouts help build you work capacity and get your mind right.

Anyway, back to that evening in the spring. I was crunched for time and I had another task that needed to get done. I had to cook dinner for my family.

I told myself laziness is out of the question so I found a way to get done what I needed to and a way to get in the extra work.

I fired up the grill on my back deck and busted out a pair of dumbbells and a drag sled. I loaded the dumbbells on the sled, dragged it across the backyard, rowed it back, then took the dumbbells off and did farmers carries around the perimeter of my property. In between rounds I would tend to the grill. It was an awesome workout followed by a great meal with my family. A win win situation!

I am not saying that rest is not important, of course it is, but laziness and self doubt will never make you better. We all have a choice, there will always be the good and the bad. I choose the good, I choose to get better, what do you choose?

ADVICE: LIFTING AND LIFE

LEARN YOUR TRADE

A long time ago, a mentor of mine told me to "learn you trade, learn it well, and you will always eat." Although I knew what he meant, I did not know, at the time, how important this was.

This lesson applies to training and to life. Both of which have come a long way for me since we had that conversation.

We all have taken things for granted at one time or another. One of the biggest things we do this with, is time. It seems like there is plenty of time when we are looking to start something new or make improvements, but truth be told, if we do not take action and are wasting time, there may not be enough.

If we are to be good at something we need to start that journey now. Not tomorrow, next week, or when we find the right help.

Take action now.

The ones in life who continuously make progress and create success, are the ones who are always learning and improving, who build upon their skills and technique.

You must be a "technician," a master of the skills at hand. Learn to master the movements to lift more weight, or hit the ball further, or whatever you goal is.

This goes for exercise, sport, your job, and your life. Learn it and learn it well.

Natural strength and talent will take you far, but a true technician will reap the benefits of health and longevity.

ARE YOU GETTING YOUR FUEL?

We cannot operate without fuel. Healthy eating habits are essential to optimize you performance. The food that you eat should give you energy to perform and decrease your recovery time. This allows your body to heal faster and be ready and stronger for the next challenge.

Protein will help build muscle. Your muscles need protein to recover from the micro tears associated with strenuous physical activity. Fats and carbohydrates will provide your body with energy. Some people are afraid of eating fats and carbohydrates because they think they will gain fat. If you eat and exercise properly, that will not happen.

You cannot eat whatever you want. For example, donuts and apple pie are not the choice you should make for carbohydrates and fat. Potatoes and avocado are much better.

Keep your eating basic. There is a reason people use the reference "meat and potatoes." It's best to stick to chicken, beef, pork, eggs, rice, sweet or white potatoes, whole wheat pasta, broccoli, green beans, asparagus, etc. When in doubt, choose the meat and potatoes.

It's best to have a consistent meal plan and you should consider hiring someone who specializes in meal plans for athletes. It will be well worth the investment, for your sports performance and for your life!

I am by no means a nutritionist but I have worked with them before and recommend that you do the same.

Here is some "food for thought"…

Fuel is NOT only for your body. You need to fuel your mind. You should be fueling your mind with positive, motivating, and inspirational stories and videos. Read positive books. Surround yourself with upbeat, likeminded people. "Mental Fuel" can help you reach the next level.

To excel and exceed your goals, you need to live and breathe the life style.

DOES THE TRAINING STOP AFTER THE WORKOUT

Our athletic program is typically three days a week. Our Powerlifitng program is typically four days a week. But both pro-grams really are seven days a week. Let me explain....

Even though the workouts are 3 or 4 days per week, a huge part of "training" is everything you do outside of the programmed workout.

I am talking about eating properly, staying positive, and not stressing out. Those who know me personally know that I have dedicated a ton of hours in my life to work and family but still al-ways find a way to get my training in. Sometimes that means not sleeping 8 hours a night and missing meals. As a competitor you need to do whatever it takes to get your practice, your training. But if missing sleep, missing meals, being stressed and being around negative energy turns into habit, the reality is you are no longer training properly.

It comes down to lifestyle. Just because you got in the workout does not mean your training is done. That's the difference between "working out" and "training." Training is what you do in and out of the gym.

I am like everyone else. Even though I love to squat, deadlift, and push my mind and body, I am not always fired up and motivated to workout. I also do not always feel like eating the healthier meal or going to bed early. It is a choice, and if you take training serious, if you take life serious, then you must realize this is a lifestyle and NOT just a workout.

Stay motivated, stay strong, and live the underground strength code of "Honesty, Integrity, Commitment and Work Ethic."

BE A POSITIVE INFLUENCE

Many of you are competitors. Competing in various sports and training hard for them. You put forth the effort to be great at what you love. Spending countless hours building up your body and skills through hard work.

All of that should not just be left behind after the game or event ends or after you retire from a great career of competing. We all need to live a strong life. Don't just be strong for the game or brave when you are training. As the late Ultimate Warrior said, "Don't just be brave under a barbell. Do it in your life!"

I want you to think about what that really means and reflect on your training and how you can apply those lessons and disciplines to your life.

I want to impact those around me in a positive way and share the lessons that I have learned along the way in my life's journey. I want others to draw influence from my life as I do from those around me. We can all learn from each other.

We can only control what we do. Find out for yourself what you are meant to do, then do it. Take action, put in your time, and share it with the world. Be a positive influence to those around you and you will be inspired to live a great life.

IS KNOWLEDGE POWER?

I often find myself putting in a lot of extra work.Working on carving out the life I want to live.It's powerful and feels awesome.It is also a bit nerve racking.

When I doubt myself and my abilities, I try to block out the negativity in my way. I change my frame of mind.I spend my time in between work, learning.I listen to podcasts and audio books.I read articles about training and business.Then I do the most important part, I take action.If you're not taking action, you are wasting time.

I remember listening to a podcast by Tony Robbins.He spoke about business strategies.Many of which can carry over into life outside of business. One point that sticks in my mind is when he said, "All of us as human beings are controlled by what we focus on." He elaborated by explaining that if you focus on the world coming to an end, if you see it and imagine it, and then you will make that your reality. It's all about your frame of mind.

Knowing this, I try and practice focusing on positive things. I focus on changing lives through strength training. I surround myself with motivated people, great coaches and of course, family. If you do not have like-minded motivated people in your life, I suggest that you surround yourself with them virtually. In today's world, with the use of social media, you can be in contact and lean from people you may never even have known existed. There is a ton of negative energy on social media, but there is also so much good too. Learn from the best and put in the work to be the best.

"Knowledge is not power. Knowledge is potential power. It all comes down to execution."-Tony Robbins

INTENT FOR THE DAY

Having a purpose for everything that you do is important if you want to achieve success. It's easy to get caught up in the many distractions that life has to offer. If you make sure that you have intent and stick to it, you will stay on the path to achieving your goals.

Apply this mindset to training. Think about your intent for the workout. Is it to move fast? Lift as much as possible? Is it to get pumped up? Know what needs to get done and do it.

It's easy to stray from the intent if you do not really have one. Every day we should all be working towards moving forward. This requires putting in the work and knowing what a distraction is, and then avoiding it. Stay focused and crush the work that you know needs to get done.

SETBACKS WON'T KEEP ME DOWN

Good times and bad times. You know the ups and the downs of life. We all go through them. It's just the way it is. What's important is, are you learning along the way? Are you finding a take-away from both the good and the bad?

I went through a major setback. This set me back with my training and more importantly, my everyday life. It forced me to make changes and that is never fun.

I also learned a great deal from this experience. I realized that I cannot just quit because it's the easier thing to do. Even though most of society would say to, "sit this one out. You've been through a lot." I figured out a different way to get things done. I learned that it's ok to get help from people. It's okay to rely on your team, your friends and your family. Sometimes you just can't do everything on your own.

I spend a great deal of my time each day, every week, every year, getting myself physically and mentally stronger. The mental strength is something that I teach my athletes every day. It's something everyone should continually be working on. This way when you are faced with the lows that life throws your way, you can persevere and come out on top. Stay strong, focused, and don't be afraid to ask for help.

INSPIRATION

I have been and continue to be inspired by so many different people and situations. There are some amazing people in my life and I'm thankful to know them. My athletes are crushing their workouts, learning and striving for excellence. I'm proud to be part of their lives. I have been to fundraisers and that feels awesome and inspiring to know that people from all different walks of life can come together and be part of something that's bigger than any one person.

Even though life throws punches at you sometimes, it doesn't mean you can call it quits. Keep your head up and things are sure to turn around. If you look around with an open mind, you will find positive inspiration. Amazing people are all around us.

I hope that you can find inspiration today. I also hope that you have goals and are working to achieve them. Sometimes it's the process that's the best part.

NEVER BE TOO BUSY TO LEARN

I often remind myself how important learning and improving is. Even if I am busy, I manage to find a way to learn something.

The old saying "learn something new every day" is true. When I was young, I thought that was ridiculous. It seemed to me something that people would say just to sound smart.

I'm older now and it makes perfect sense. There is opportunity all around to learn something new. I learn from reading on article or watching a video. I learn from coaching my athletes and working with prospects. I also learn from making mistakes and putting myself out there in uncomfortable challenging places and situations. Sometimes it feels like if I just look around, the answers to learning how to improve myself are all around me.

Something that I found helpful and can help you, is to reflect back on your day and recognize the situations which you can learn from. Not all learning needs to be behind a desk with your face in a text book, or sitting in a chair listening to a lecture. Learn from real life experiences that you are having and you will be on the path to self improvement and real life happiness.

ARE YOU MAKING AN IMPACT?

There are so many challenges that we all face on a day to day basis. Life has its way of making things difficult.

It is very common to dread Mondays. So many people do not like getting up on Monday morning to start their work week. There was a time period in my life that I felt the same way. During this time, I was wasting so much energy being negative and I didn't even realize it. Eventually I changed my mind set, which allowed me to change my circumstances and in turn, change my life.

I found a way to draw from and share positivity from others. And this has made a positive impact on my life. Now when I lie down at night, I can feel good about my day. I know that I gave 100% effort to the things that I was involved in. Doing this is not easy. Every day, like everyone else in the world, I face difficulties that challenge me and test my will to being positive but having the right attitude surrounding yourself with positive influences and cutting out what's negative, can make a world of difference.

"Don't just be a leader, be a leader for the leaders."-Warrior

DO NOT JUST DREAM YOUR LIFE AWAY

What do you dream of? Not when you're asleep, but your passions. What are your passions?

Knowing your answers to these questions is important because when you recognize what you love, it will spark something very inspiring inside of you. Having this knowledge about yourself is powerful.

But if you never pursue you passions, all you are doing is dreaming. Having hopes and dreams is great, but taking action is what matters most.

I know this first hand. Being able to coach athletes and change peoples' lives through strength training is my passion. When I realized this, it changed my life.

One of my mentors told me, "People like us are put on this Earth to help people be strong." Having him recognize this inspired me big time. It felt like a green light for me to go against what was "normal" for me, and follow my dreams.

This is what I want you to do. Follow your passions and live the life that you were meant to live. Trust in your heart and follow your passions.Even if it makes no sense to those around you. Your actions will inspire others. Do not just go through life being a dreamer. Learn to live those dreams.

BE CONFIDENT

I hope that you are charging hard towards being a better you and attacking your goals. It is easier said than done to have goals and actually achieve them. I like to think big and sometimes I dream bigger than I can handle at the time. By dreaming big I learn a great deal about what I am capable of. By setting goals, I stay committed.

The reality is, we are all capable of doing anything as long as we commit to actually doing it. One of the most powerful things that you can have in your life is confidence.

The power of the mind is extraordinary and when you believe that you will accomplish something, you will. When you make excuses to yourself, you lose confidence. You may fool other people on the outside, but deep down you know if you are doing what needs to be done. Don't fool yourself, believe in yourself.

We all define what a great life is differently. That's the beauty. Life is what you make it be. We all deserve to live a great life, but that's a choice, not a rule. I can promise that even though you will be challenged, if you put in the work, you will feel good. That starts with a strong and confident mind.

VALUABLE LIFE LESSONS

Many valuable life lessons can be learned in sports, strength training, and really any fitness journey.

I want to share a few of these key things that I have learned and will help bring you value.

You cannot just think and dream about the things that you want. You must be dedicated to the work in order to reach your goals.

Strength come from your body and your mind

You must be the one who builds yourself up. Don't use the short comings of others to boost your ego. That gets you nowhere.

Take responsibility for your actions. At the end of the day, you get what you earn.

Believe in yourself

Always be humble

WORK HARD, FEEL GOOD